Emotional Intel

The Mindfulness Guide To Mastering Your Emotions, Getting Ahead And Improving Your Life

Your Free Gift

As a way of thanking you for the purchase, I'd like to offer you a complimentary gift:

- **5 Pillar Life Transformation Checklist:** This short book is about life transformation, presented in bit size pieces for easy implementation. I believe that without such a checklist, you are likely to have a hard time implementing anything in this book and any other thing you set out to do religiously and sticking to it for the long haul. It doesn't matter whether your goals relate to weight loss, relationships, personal finance, investing, personal development, improving communication in your family, your overall health, finances, improving your sex life, resolving issues in your relationship, fighting PMS successfully, investing, running a successful business, traveling etc. With a checklist like this one, you can bet that anything you do will seem a lot easier to implement until the end. Therefore, even if you don't continue reading this book, at least read the one thing that will help you in every other aspect of your life. Grab your copy now by clicking/tapping here or simply enter http://bit.ly/2fantonfreebie into your browser. Your life will never be the same again (if you implement what's in this book), I promise.

PS: I'd like your feedback. If you are happy with this book, please leave a review on Amazon.

Introduction

Jason is a 30-year-old married man who married the love of his life and now has two kids: a boy 'Daniel' aged 3 and a nine-month-old girl 'Sarah'. Although the society labels mothers as more patient beings, it is Jason who manages his kids calmly and stays peaceful amidst their tantrums. Whenever Daniel throws a tantrum or behaves in an undesirable manner, Jason is the one who tends to him and calms him down in an assertive manner.

Not only is Jason a pro in handling his kids, he is also great when it comes to disagreements with his wife 'Jessica'. Jessica is hot-tempered, so they argue often, but are always able to resolve them since Jason never reacts rashly. Moreover, he has always enough time for his family and juggles both, professional and personal lives well since he can maintain a balance between the two easily.

He is quite an ambitious person and has an ultimate goal of becoming the CEO of the company he works for. Currently, he is the head of the marketing department and is one of the best employees the company has ever had. Although his boss is quite an obstinate man, Jason gets his way with him as he is open to change, is flexible, and knows how to handle people well. He never loses hope and has a positive outlook towards life, which is why he has been successful in maintaining peace both at home and in the office. Yes, he does go through difficult times and loses his calm at times, but he knows how to manage it and does not let others be negatively affected by it.

Now you may probably be wondering that Jason is somewhat a superhero because such men may seem rare nowadays. Nope, you're wrong! He is a normal human being who has amazingly high emotional intelligence (EQ). Yes, the reason behind his beautiful life and a composed character is his high EQ and it isn't something he was born with. It is something he built and nurtured over the years. If he can do it, so can you.

But how can you improve your EQ? What do you need to do to accomplish this goal? Well, this is where this helpful guide comes in handy. Created as a complete emotional intelligence guide, this book provides you with proven strategies to master your emotions and enhance your EQ to become amazingly confident.

I hope you enjoy it!

Table of Contents

Understanding Emotional Intelligence

Emotional intelligence (EI) is also referred to as emotional quotient (EQ) and is your capacity to understand and realize your emotions as well as those of others, so you can distinguish different feelings easily and label them correctly.

Being emotionally intelligence basically means that you are able to identify the different emotions as you experience them promptly and have the ability to manage them well. On the other hand, if you lack this ability, you aren't able to identify the different emotions you may be experiencing and you get confused by the concoction of emotions brewing up inside you. As you cannot understand an emotion as it takes place, you aren't able to successfully manage it as well. Instead of channeling the emotion appropriately, you express it in an undesirable manner. Let us simplify this description with an example.

If you are hurt by someone you love, you start feeling angry and frustrated. However, since your EQ is quite low, you aren't able to understand why you feel a certain way, or may not even be able to realize the true emotion and may take it to be sadness or depression. When you become very angry, you may start shouting at someone or you may even throw a big tantrum in your house, storming at anyone and everyone who comes in front of you.

As opposed to this, if you did have a high EQ, you wouldn't react this way. You would spot your anger and frustration as soon as it kicks in and would look for calmer and rational ways to channel it. You may sit somewhere quiet and practice deep breathing as you feel your anger increase and subside inside you or you may write about that negative experience that infuriated you and let go of your fury through your words. Since you have control over your emotions, you did not target any innocent being with your rage and calmed yourself down in the most relaxed manner.

Similarly, if you spotted your ex-boyfriend with his new girlfriend in the mall and became jealous on seeing them walk hand in hand, you may go up to them and say something rude to both of them if your EQ is low. On the contrary, if you did have a remarkably high EQ, you would probably not interact with them if you knew you still were hurt and had not forgiven your ex. Instead of lashing at them, you would leave that place and then take out your negative feelings in a calm way such as meditation or journaling your thoughts. Hence, having emotional intelligence is a great quality that ensures you keep your cool and use your energies in the right manner.

Let us look at what emotional intelligence entails

What Does Emotional Intelligence Encompass?

Daniel Goleman, a renowned American psychologist created a framework encompassing five components that best describe emotional intelligence.

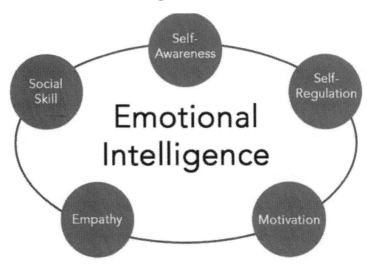

Self-Awareness: Also referred to as emotional awareness, self-awareness is the ability to recognize your emotions as well as those of people around you. Emotional intelligence makes you aware of what's going on inside you and spot an emotion as soon as it occurs. It makes you comprehend your emotions, which enables you to gradually tame them and get control over them. Self-awareness not only helps you take charge of your emotions, but it also makes you confident as you know you won't let your emotions get the better of you and you trust your intuition. The ability to be consciously aware of your emotions also helps you become honest with yourself and analyze yourself in the most honest manner. You become aware of your weaknesses and strengths, know your short-comings and know how to overcome your weaknesses and improve your strengths.

Self-Regulation: Self-regulation refers to the ability to manage and control your emotions, so that they never rule you. This ability gives you the power to regulate the different negative emotions residing inside you and let go of them with time. When you can manage your emotions well, you avoid making careless and impulsive decisions. You always think before you act which makes you composed and poised. Additionally, as you can regulate your emotions well, you manage the tendency of saying yes to anyone who approaches you for a favor and resist becoming a people-pleaser.

Motivation: Motivation is another prominent element of EQ. As you cope with your negative emotions successfully, you keep disappointments and pessimism at bay from yourself, which helps you stay motivated to achieve your goals. You can easily defer the instant gratification and immediate results in order to achieve long-term success. Since you are highly motivated, you are productive as well, which increases your chances of success.

Empathy: Often regarded as the second most significant component of emotional intelligence, empathy refers to the capacity to recognize and comprehend the needs, wants, feelings, and opinions of people around you. High EQ increases your empathy which gives you the power to recognize the pains and miseries of those around you quickly. As you are empathetic towards others, you are able to manage relationships well and have good listening skills.

Social Skills: another important element of EQ is social skills. When you can manage yourself successfully amongst others, have good listening skills, are confident and empathetic, you are definitely able to interact well with people. Your excellent social skills help you become a team player as well as a team leader.

Emotional intelligence does not only make you control your emotions, but it helps you reach your full potential and be the best of yourself. It is often compared with IQ and many people used to believe that it was the latter that determined your success or failure in life. Let us explore the differences between the two and find out which of the two is more important for you to succeed in life.

Difference Between IQ And EQ

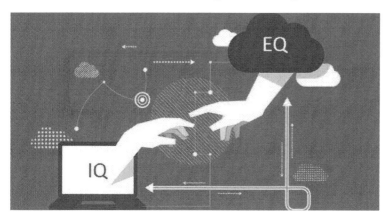

While EQ is your capacity to recognize, assess and manage your emotions or those experienced by others, IQ (intelligence quotient) on the other hand is a measure of your intelligence and is a score extracted from one of the standardized tests created to assess your intelligence. Your IQ gives an idea of how intelligent you are and is considered as a good measure of your learning capacity and the ability to understand different information, process it, and apply it to different situations. On the contrary, EQ expresses your ability to evaluate, assess, realize, and manage emotions.

Another different between the two is that IQ proves to be helpful in challenging tasks and gives you the ability to connect different cues together and reach conclusions. Moreover, it comes in handy when you conduct research on something. On the other hand, your EQ helps you settle in a group and become a team player. If you continue to improve your EQ, you can emerge as the group and team leader as well. It also ensures successful relations, great collaborative capacities and helps you empower others.

Now that we have a better understanding of these two, which is more important? Your IQ is a good indicator of how intelligent you are, but your intelligence is not the only determinant of your success in life. You may be able to analyze a situation well and make informed decisions, but your IQ does not give you the power to influence others, form successful and profitable relations with them, and use your energies, efforts, and emotions in the most appropriate manner. It is your EQ that gives you this ability, which is why it is considered to be a more viable indicator of success in your life.

Success is defined in a number of ways by different people. For you it might be to live happily with your family and ensure that your children get the best education and opportunities in life. On the other hand, someone else may define it in monetary terms and consider themselves successful only when they become a billionaire. In whatever way you define it, you need a few important elements to become successful in both, your personal and professional life.

First, you need to be aware of your goals, which is only possible when you know yourself better and are able to understand your emotional needs, and you can only manage your emotions and meet your emotional needs when you have a high EQ.

Secondly, you need to stick to your goals and have the grit to actualize your objectives. Grit is a combination of perseverance, resilience, stubbornness, optimism, confidence, and creativity. You can only persevere in difficult times when you can control yourself and focus on what's importance. You can become resilient and stubborn only when you have the ability to stay true to your mission and overcome temptations. You can become confident, creative, and optimistic when you can manage your negativities easily and overpower them. And all of this is only possible when you have emotional intelligence.

Thirdly, you need to form good relationships with people to make good use of attractive opportunities in your professional life and you need to make peace at home with your loved ones to live a beautiful life. Both these things are only possible when you have control over your emotions, are empathetic towards others, have compassion for them and have good social skills. This again is possible only by developing emotional intelligence.

This means that your IQ does signify your intelligence and shrewdness, it does not in any way define that you will be successful in life. On the other hand, if you are emotionally intelligence, your chances of success are quite high. This isn't just a theory, but has been proven by studies that show that having EQ boosts entrepreneurial potential, success in career, relationship satisfaction and leadership potential.

Can EQ Be Developed Or Is It An Inborn Ability?

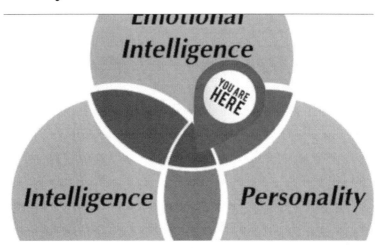

Your ability to spot emotions and manipulate them is mainly influenced by your genes and early childhood experiences, and it tends to remain stable with time. However, this does not mean you cannot change and improve your EQ. You can certainly improve your EQ. A study also shows that your EQ tends to experience a <u>slight increase as you age</u>.

However, to ensure your EQ is high enough to make you successful, you need to put in hard work and effort on your own, and this is where the mindfulness strategy comes in handy. It is one of the best and proven techniques to enhance your emotional quotient. Let us learn more about mindfulness and how you can tap into it to improve your EQ.

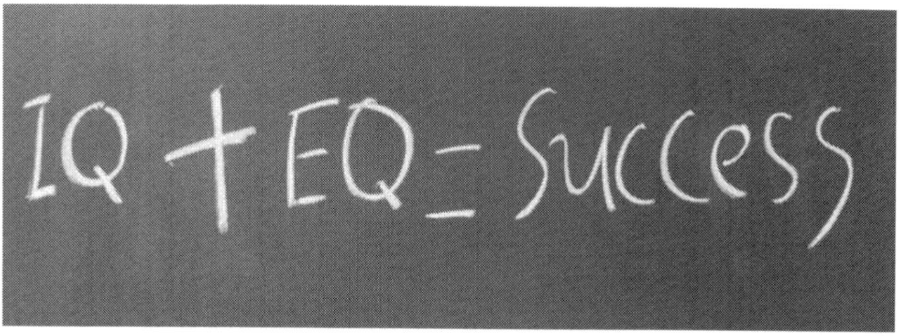
IQ + EQ = Success

Strategies To Increase EQ

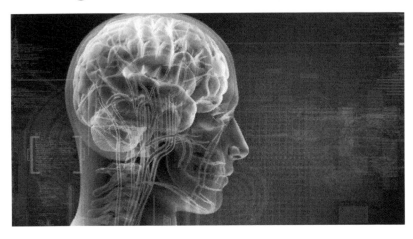

Now that you have a basic idea of what EQ is and how it can do wonders for you, let us find out the strategies you need to implement to improve your EQ.

Improve Non-Verbal Communication

Albert Merhabian, who is the professor Emeritus of Psychology at the UCLA found out from his research that a staggering 55 percent of your routine communication with others is the result of your body language, about 38 percent is para-linguistic which means it is done by your pauses, tones, pace etc. and only 7 percent is pertinent to the words you actually speak.

The bottom line is that your body language is undoubtedly an incredibly powerful and effective component of how you communicate. The way you move, stand, tilt your head and pace yourself speaks a lot about your confidence, emotional stability and resolute to others.

For example, there are two people standing on the stage in front of you: one with his head tilted to the side, arms crossed, legs closed, and shoulders narrowed and the other standing firmly with shoulders open and head held high, looking directly at you. Which one seems more poised, self-assured and emotionally confident to you? Of course, the second one. And why is that? Because his body language is stronger than that of the first one and reflects his confidence and emotional intelligence. He seems sure of himself and knows how to face people as well as manage them, whereas the first person seems scared and timid. This simple example shows that your body language actually communicates a lot more to the people about your EQ than you think and it is an important strategy to improve your emotional quotient. Not only does this strategy helps you improve your body language so you communicate successfully with others, but it also helps you read the body language of others and understand their emotions and feelings, which helps you understand them and use them to your benefit.

This means that you need to pay attention to your body language and find out what to improve so you convey the right message to your audience.

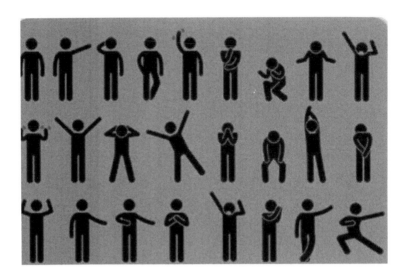

Become Assertive

"Being who we are requires that we can talk openly about things that are important to us, that we take a clear position on where we stand on important emotional issues, and that we clarify the limits of what is acceptable and tolerable to us in a relationship." - Harriet Lerner

There does come time in your life when you need to set appropriate boundaries for others, so they know where you stand. Being emotionally strong and intelligent doesn't mean you need to only understand how others feel and be compassionate with them even if that means giving them advantage over you. In fact, it means to be well aware of every situation that takes place and handle oneself and others in the most suitable manner. Being assertive is an important and helpful strategy to improve your emotional intelligence as it helps you say no to others without feeling remorseful, allows you to set your priorities, get what you paid for as well as protect yourself from harm and duress.

For instance, you are hired as an accountant in a firm. Your boss is happy with your work and to please him, you are always ready to do favors for him, as you fear being assertive may make you lose your job. He senses your fear and burdens you with extra work pertinent to the marketing and HR department of the firm. You are supposed to leave work at 5pm every day, but you stay until 8 daily. You know what is happening with you and it is causing too much pressure on you but since you are not assertive, you don't do something about the situation.

On the other hand, if you had high emotional intelligence, you would handle this scenario in a different manner. You may do a favor for your boss once or twice, but then you'll let him know that you have been hired as an accountant only and you can consider doing extra chores only if you'll get paid extra for it. You need to say it in a confident but gentle manner. This ensures that your boss doesn't take advantage of your courteousness and knows that you aren't a people pleaser, so he needs to behave well with you.

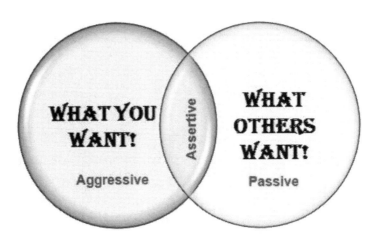

Mindfulness

Of all the strategies discovered to increase emotional intelligence, mindfulness is arguably the most beneficial, effective and successful one. It is often regarded as the foundation of emotional intelligence. Mindfulness basically refers to being present in the moment you are experiencing right now. Jon Kabat-Zinn, one of the pioneers of mindfulness meditation and the creator of Mindfulness-based Stress Reduction program describes mindfulness as paying attention to your present moment purposely and nonjudgmentally. This means that you need to be focused on the present moment and need to be aware of everything happening with and around you right now, but in a gentle, unbiased, and calm manner. While this may seem like something, you already do, in reality it is not.

Mindfulness is not just doing routine tasks. Our hectic routines have made us sort of robotic. Whenever you get a task, your aim is to complete it as soon as possible. If you were eating food, you would do it quickly so you could move on to working. If you were making a presentation, you'd try your best to finish it as fast as there is another task lined up for you. While you do things hurriedly, you fail to experience the act completely. You aren't aware of how every grain of rice feels in your mouth or what emotions go through your mind as you work on the presentation.

Moreover, when you do spot something, your perception of it is most probably a biased one. If your experience with a situation or element has been positive in the past, your perception of it now will be positive too even if the current scenario is slightly negative. You can never be truly nonjudgmental about something unless and until you learn to be mindful.

One major reason why you cannot concentrate on things happening in and around you is because you aren't fully aware of yourself. You don't know who you are, what you want, what emotions you experience with each passing moment, why you feel the way you feel and what you must do to live a better life. You do not dwell in the present because you are either too concerned about improving your future or you are too busy contemplating on and stressing about things that happened in the past. These concerns make you forgetful of the present and everything it holds within: you, your life, your feelings, your loved ones, and all the moments you are letting go of.

Being forgetful makes you miss on the little pleasures of life and makes you disregard all that you have now. It also makes you ignorant of your own emotions. You may be feeling upset and stressed, but the worry of completing a project on time and submitting it the next day makes you push yourself harder without paying attention to your feelings. This makes negative emotions build up inside you and then one fine day, you take the storm out in the most irrational manner on someone when you can no longer keep it inside you. It is okay if you have been feeling this way and behaving in a certain manner. We all go through such scenarios. However, what's important is that you need to improve yourself and your emotional intelligence if you truly want to achieve any of your goals and this is where mindfulness comes in useful.

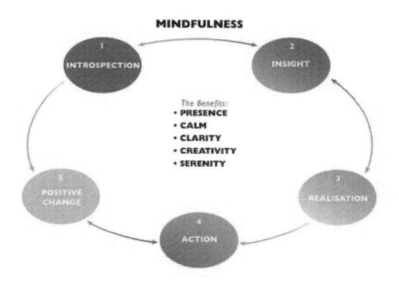

Mindfulness makes you aware

When you become mindful, you start to become aware of everything that occurs inside you as well as around you. Mindfulness teaches you to focus on your thoughts and be aware of them, as it is your thoughts that induce different emotions in you that produce certain behaviors. For instance, you think someone hates you and you feel sad and have negative emotions towards him or her. This makes you rude at that person. Similarly, if you experience a happy thought, you are going to behave positively.

Normally, you are so engaged in multiple activities and thinking processes at the same time that you fail to fully recognize the different positive and negative thoughts you experience. Since you are cognizant of the right and wrong thoughts, you tend to ruminate on the unhealthy ones and act upon them. This is why you are unable to realize your emotions easily and manage them. However, by becoming mindful, you learn the art of becoming consciously aware of your thoughts as they enter and leave your mind, so you know which ones to keep and filter.

When you become fully aware of things, you are able to think straight and make the right decisions.

Mindfulness makes you unbiased

Mindfulness teaches you to perceive and analyze things as they happen and individually, so you don't assess a situation judgmentally. When you take things for what they are, your perspective of situations and things improves and this helps you tackle scenarios from different approaches easily. Moreover, this makes you compassionate towards others, as you are able to understand their sentiments and comprehend their feelings in an unbiased manner.

Mindfulness improves your emotional well-being

Various documented research studies have shown that mindfulness relieves anxiety, stress, and depression, improves your focus and your emotional well-being. Mark Coleman, a renowned mindfulness teacher states that mindfulness makes you attentive of yourself and your surroundings in the most nonjudgmental and gentle way and this makes you tap into your emotional side and stabilize it. He has given mindfulness training to over 3,000 employees at Google, so they can enhance their emotional intelligence and improve their productivity at work and even in other situations.

Mindfulness makes you happy

Not only does mindfulness instill consciousness and fairness in you, but it also makes you happy and peaceful. Latest research by Matt Killingsworth, a researcher from Harvard shows that we are happy when we are fully aware of the present moment. This makes us focus on the now and be aware of it and all the blessings it has. When we are happy and live in the present, we slowly let go of our worries attached to the past or future and this helps us attain inner peace.

Daily Life Examples

Let us look at daily life examples of how mindfulness improves your emotional intelligence

Example 1: You have been selected to be in a project management team, but you have issues with one of the team members. You don't get along well since he has a bad habit of calling you weird names. If you aren't mindful of your emotions and thoughts, you would probably give in to the thought of shouting back at him, abusing him or maybe even hitting him. However, if you cultivate mindfulness in yourself, you will identify and recognize the different negative emotions as you experience and will know how to calm them down. In addition, you will assess your colleague's behavior nonjudgmentally and will understand that for him to be that negative then he is the one with the problem and not you. Once you have this understanding, his comments will affect not affect you as much.

Example 2: Your spouse earns more than you do and this has been creating rifts between you and your spouse for a couple of months. Whenever your spouse discusses financial matters with you, you feel they are blaming you for earning less and you start quarrelling with them without listening to them completely. You aren't able to understand the real scenario and understand your spouse's concern because you feel guilty for earning less. Since you aren't fully aware of your emotions, you blame everything on your spouse.

On the other hand, if you are mindful of your emotions and thoughts, you would first try to make peace with the fact that you are earning less and it is nobody else's fault. You would focus on separating your negative thoughts from the positive ones and identify the real cause of your anger. This would slowly help you eliminate negativity from your mind and you would start to focus on things individually, which would make you pay attention to your spouse's talk and comprehend their concern.

Example 3: You lose your job, which was the main source of livelihood for you and your family. This traumatizes you and you become highly depressed. You feel there's nothing you can do now and instead of looking for other opportunities, you fall in the depression trap. You waste your time and energy thinking on why this stressful event happened and this makes you ill tempered. If you were mindful, you would tackle this situation quite differently. Instead of thinking how it happened and how it would ruin your future, you would think of how you can counter it. Since you are aware of the present moment, you would take a moment to count many of your blessings despite losing a job. This calms your mind and makes you think rationally. Once you are relaxed, you would think of all the ways to find another better job so you can get out of the financial crisis and improve things. Instead of letting the negative situation overpower you, you would use your ability to think positively to fix that situation and eventually improve it.

By becoming mindful, you are able to harmonize your emotions, get better insight into yourself and your needs, understand your feelings, filter negative thoughts, think positively, and improve yourself for the better. Therefore, you not only become emotionally strong and intelligent, but you enhance every aspect of your personality. This is why mindfulness is considered as the best way to enhance your EQ.

There are several other strategies to improve your emotional intelligence but these three are undoubtedly the best ones, especially mindfulness because it helps you shape every tiny aspect of your personality and develop a strong, influential and calm persona that affects everyone positively. Now that you have a basic understanding of these strategies, let us find out how you need to implement them.

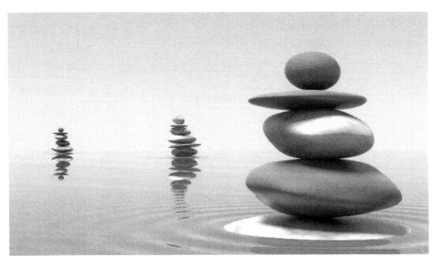

Applying Daily Mindfulness Practice To Increase EQ

Becoming mindful of your thoughts, feelings, and emotions is a skill that takes time to develop, but practice, persistence, and hard work is all you need. Here is what you need to do to attain complete mindfulness of yourself and surroundings.

Exercise 1: Mindful Breathing

According to Thich Nhat Hanh, the first step to becoming mindful is to become mindful of your breathing. You need to simply identify your in-breath and out-breath as you inhale and exhale. As you breathe, you need to become conscious of your breathing and recognize your in and out breaths as you take them. To do that, it is important you sit somewhere peaceful so you can stay alert and focus entirely on your breathing without becoming distracted.

After you have settled down in a quiet place, just focus on your breathing movement and keep your thoughts concentrated on your inhalation and exhalation only. This makes you become fully attentive of your breath and nothing else. Soon, you will find all the mental discourse coming to a halt and you'll find a sort of stillness settling in your mind. You wouldn't have made any conscious effort to achieve that, just focusing on your breathing helps you accomplish this calmness. When this happens, your thoughts wander nowhere but become grounded in the present. You start to enjoy this practice as it makes you feel serene and peaceful.

Remember to breathe very naturally. If your in-breath is four seconds long then don't prolong it to five seconds. You don't have to make a deliberate effort to breathe deeply, you just need to focus on your breathing and with time, it will slow down.

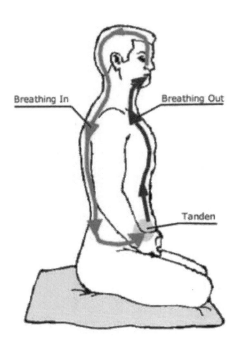

Improve Your Concentration

You must also try to follow your breath from the moment it starts until the time it ends. For instance, if you just inhaled, then follow your in-breath until you exhale the breath. Stay with your breath from the time you inhale until the time you exhale. This improves your concentration and makes you stay with your breathing movements. This practice is important as it teaches you to become fully involved in a practice as you do.

How often have you drank tea mindfully and enjoyed every sip of the concoction of water and tealeaves? Not quite often, right. This is because your mind wanders to other worries every time and you aren't able to live in the moment. The practice of deliberately following your breath helps you live in the moment and experience each moment as it occurs. If you do become distracted by a thought, you need to gently bring your attention back to your breathing. Remember to be soft and nice with yourself as being harsh doesn't do you any good.

Do this practice several times in a day and at least for five minutes each time. In about two weeks, you will be able to concentrate on your breathing easily and will be able to become mindful of other activities you do as well.

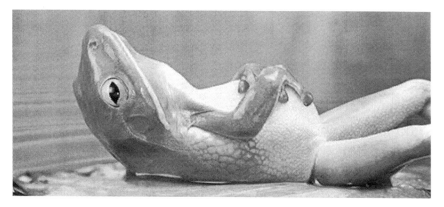

Exercise 2: Becoming Mindful Of Your Body

Once you start to gain better awareness of your breathing, you need to enhance your awareness of your body. For that, you need to start by breathing naturally and then bring your focus to your body. As you breathe in and out, you need to start becoming conscious of your body. Focus on how you feel as you breathe in and out, how your abdomen moves, how your pelvic muscles stretch and contract, your tummy muscles expand and the sensation that you experience in your entire body.

This exercise unites your body and mind, and brings the two in one place. Unity of your mind and body is crucial for EQ.

Doing this exercise daily helps you gain better control of your body and mind, and make the most of them.

Exercise 3: Walking Meditation

Once you start to become better at breathing consciously and becoming mindful of your body, you need to move on to walking meditation. This requires you to meditate while you walk. To practice it, you need to walk in a quiet, serene place and focus on your breathing and body movements as you take a step forward. Try to become aware of yourself as you walk. You may falter at first but don't worry, practice will help you get there. Stick to this practice for at least ten minutes and within a day or two, you will be able to practice walking meditation. It is an enjoyable experience for you as it brings your mind and body in unison and makes you feel alive and present in the moment. This helps you gain self-awareness as you do any task.

Once you perfect simple walking meditation, you need to practice mindfulness meditation with other tasks, such as eating, drinking, cleaning, writing and so on. For instance, if you are eating, start by becoming mindful of your breathing and body movements and then take a bite. As you take a bite, chew it slowly and feel it move through your throat and inside your body. This way you let your thoughts stay focused in the act and prevent them from wandering anywhere else.

Quite soon, you will do everything in a state of mindfulness and will be fully aware of yourself, your emotions and feelings as you do anything. And when that happens, your emotional quotient multiplies by manifolds.

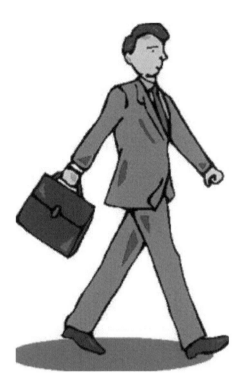

Quick 10 Minute Mindfulness Meditation Practice

The exercises discussed above train you to make mindfulness a constant part of your life. Here is a quick practice extracted from the exercises above that you can practice anywhere and at any time to realign your thoughts and get hold of yourself.

1. Lie down or sit in a quiet place for at least five to ten minutes.

2. As you settle in the place, you need to pay attention to your breath coming in and going out of the inner lining of your nostrils.

3. Relax yourself and focus only on your in-breath and out-breath and nothing else.

4. You may find some thoughts entering your awareness. If that happens, you need to softly bring your focus back to your nostrils and the air moving in and out of them.

5. In about five minutes, you will find yourself becoming calmer. This may take longer if you aren't a regular practitioner of mindfulness meditation.

6. Once you find calmness settling inside you and your thoughts slowing down, you need to start to focus on your body. Try to identify and notice any feelings you experience and then label each one as you experience it. Make sure not to work out the reason behind the existence of those feelings, just name each as you feel it.

7. As you experience and name a feeling, you need to tell yourself that emotions are complex to handle and the best way to manage them effectively is not to give them extra importance. You need to just acknowledge the emotion and let it pass out of your body on its own without giving it any undue attention. For instance, if you just had a fight with your best friend and you're mad at them, you need to acknowledge your anger and then let it subside and move out of your body by simply focusing on your breathing. This may seem impossible right now, but when you do it, you'll realize how wonderful this technique actually is.

You can practice this technique at any time of the day and at any place. For instance, if you find yourself becoming envious of your colleague in your workplace who just got promoted whereas you were expecting to receive that accolade, you could excuse yourself and go to the toilet. Sit or stand and practice this simple exercise and within minutes, you will find the envy vanishing away from your mind and body.

If you had a big argument with your partner and you fear the fight may end your relationship, you need to just get out of the situation and go take a stroll out in the open and practice this technique. Similarly, this practice can easily be done anywhere, you just need to have the commitment and drive for it. Make it a regular part of your life and very soon, there will come a time when you will manage every situation, every problem and every person like a pro.

Improving Body Language To Boost Your EQ

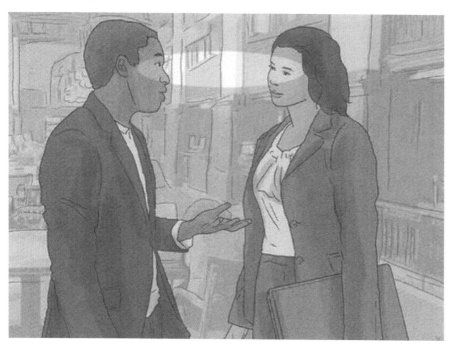

Improving your body language plays a monumental role in giving a big boost to your emotional intelligence. When you portray yourself as a strong, confident, and influential person, people are likely to pay attention to you and eventually pay heed to what you say. Let us find out how you can make your body language work in your favor.

Warm up with a high power pose

According to Harvard researcher Amy Cuddy, there are certain body poses known as high power poses that boost the levels of testosterone in your body, which is a hormone associated with boosting confidence. Exercising those poses daily helps your confidence increase and as your confidence improves, your ability to influence those around you changes as well. Additionally, your high self-confidence makes you sure of yourself, helping you manage your emotions easily.

One of the best high power poses is the superman pose. Stand straight with your shoulders open and place your hands on your hips. Keep your head high and look straight. Do it for about five minutes daily and soon your confidence levels will increase.

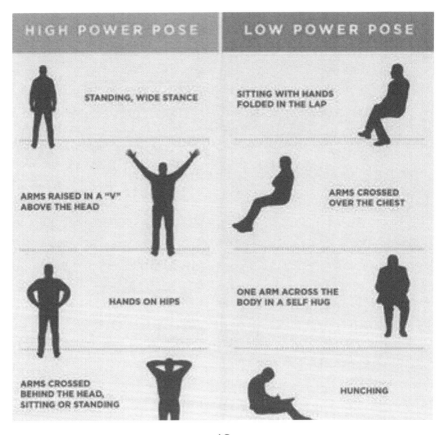

Maintain direct eye contact

Your eye contact plays a huge impact on the ones you communicate with. A study carried out in 1989 proved that maintaining direct eye contact with someone could even make them fall in love with you. When you look someone directly in the eye, you tell him or her that you are completely self-assured and you know what you are saying. When your gaze stays strong, they can feel your confidence and listen to you. In addition, a softer gaze is a good way to show empathy to others and make them feel you care. Your eyes speak a lot more than you think which is why you need to make good use of them when interacting with people.

When you need to convince someone and make an impression on them, you need to look them straight in the eye with sheer confidence. However, if you need to show someone you care, you need to soften your gaze by making your eyes seem less stern.

Talk using your hands

Using hand gestures while talking is a good way to convey your message to your audience professionally. Expressing yourself with hand gestures reflects your confidence and poise.

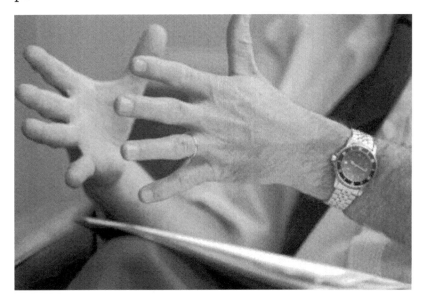

Show your audience you're listening to them

To improve your social skills, you need to interact with people and pay close attention to them. A common characteristic observed in almost all charismatic personalities, including Steve Jobs and Oprah Winfrey is that they pay attention to their audience and actually listen to them. To improve your social skills, you need to let people feel that you care for them and a good tip to do this is to take interest in their talk. Put your phone on silent or vibration mode when you enter a big gathering and reduce your temptation to do anything, such as check your watch or phone when someone speaks to you. When people know you are care for them, they eventually pay attention to you and return you the favor.

Mirroring Technique

You need to build a good rapport with someone to inspire and influence them. And 'mirroring' is a good technique for this. It requires you to imitate another person's action, body language, and behaviors. For instance, if someone you want to connect with is shaking their right leg, you could do that as well and within minutes, they will feel close and familiar to you.

Make these strategies a part of your routine to take your EQ to the next level.

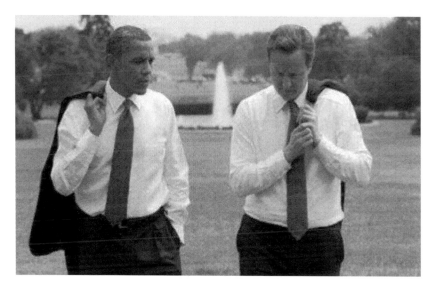

Being Assertive To Improve Your EQ

Having the ability to say no to others when needed is extremely important to stay emotionally strong and influential. Here are some practical tips to become assertive.

Standing your ground

The first thing you need to do to become assertive is to stand your ground when you make a decision. For instance, if you say NO once you have made up your mind do not budge from your stance. To ensure you do that, you need to constantly think that you matter the most to yourself. This will motivate you to stand your ground.

Present proof

If you want to portray yourself as the authority figure and let people know you have command over a subject, you must research it well so you know every detail attached to it and you must back it with documented, solid proof. This lets people you know what you're saying and have full knowledge of what you're saying.

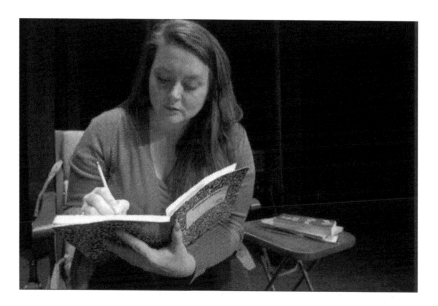

Talk with confidence

If you have been practicing high power poses and are working on improving your body language, your confidence will start to increase. When you gain confidence, you automatically become assertive too.

Remove Guilt

Being assertive and firm can be quite tough, particularly if you have been a people pleaser or passive most of your life. Saying no to someone may be accompanied by a strong guilt at first. You may feel bad for saying no to someone, but remember being assertive is essential for your emotional well-being. In order to stay emphatic and forceful on the decisions you take, you need to let go of the guilt residing inside you. A good way to do that is by becoming mindful and practicing deep breathing regularly.

Take a deep breath in and focus on the guilt inside you. Hold your breath for about five seconds and acknowledge the power of your guilty feeling. Next, you need to exhale and count up to five. As you do that, imagine your guilt getting out of your system as well. You could give a color to your guilt and as you exhale, picture that ball of guilt moving out of you. Doing this practice on a regular basis soon makes you guilt-free and consequently assertive.

It is important to practice these strategies daily to perfect them and make the most of them.

Developing EQ To Increase Your Self-Confidence

There exists a strong relationship between your emotional intelligence and confidence. Let us find out how a higher EQ improves your confidence and how you can develop it by using mindfulness.

Relationship Between EQ And Self-Confidence

When you are sure of your emotions and can handle them successfully, you become positive of yourself. You know that you have the ability to control a situation like a pro and you can present your demands and needs to others easily. This automatically elevates your confidence and makes you sure of yourself. You have that can-do attitude because of your ability to manage yourself and others. Hence, emotional intelligence and self-confidence are directly proportional to one another. A study focused on the effects of motivation, confidence and emotional intelligence proved that as your EQ increases, your self-confidence rises as well.

Moreover, research carried out by the Carnegie Institute of Technology shows that around 85 percent of your financial skills are due to your ability to communicate strongly, negotiate with others, and lead them and your personality. These qualities improve as your EQ improves and when your emotional intelligence improves so does your confidence.

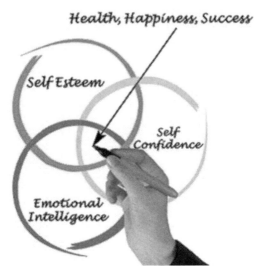

How Mindfulness Increases Your EQ And Confidence?

Now that you have basic understanding of the relationship between EQ and self-confidence, let us focus on how you can improve both these skills with the help of mindfulness.

The following example will give you a clearer idea of how beautifully mindfulness affects your EQ and self-confidence.

Anne is a 27-year-old woman who isn't sure of herself and is a big people pleaser. If someone does not respond to her messages, she feels she has done something wrong to upset them. She never trusts her decisions and lacks the confidence to believe in herself.

By learning mindfulness, Anne can learn the trick to pause the negative thought streams she experiences 24/7 whenever she wants. As these negative, self-limiting thoughts diminish, she will have better control of her emotions and will become sure of herself, her abilities, and her decisions. This will make her self-esteem and self-confidence automatically improve.

If mindfulness can help her get out of her shell of lack of belief and low self-image, it can do the same for you. Here's what you need to do to achieve this goal.

Supply your mind and body with small doses of mindfulness

You don't need to hit your yoga mat each time to practice mindfulness. You can do it anytime and anywhere, you just need to have the will for it. Adding small doses of this wonderful tactic is the perfect way to attain a calmer and peaceful state of mind. To do that, you need to do the following:

1. Focus on your breathing, especially when you feel stressed.

2. Let your thoughts flow through your mind without holding on to them or ruminating on them. Thoughts are designed to enter and leave your mind, but it is you who holds them. Just let them flow out of your mind as they enter and don't judge them.

3. Whenever you feel unsure of yourself, you need to bring your thoughts back to the present and take interest in the activity you are doing. This will make you dwell in the present and let go of negativity rooted inside you.

Routine practice of these steps will boost your EQ and your self-belief.

Developing EQ To Increase Your Self-Confidence And Leadership Skills

Your emotional intelligence has a direct impact on your leadership skills. The more emotional intelligence you are the higher your chances of becoming a good leader. Let us explore this relationship further and teach you how to use mindfulness to build these skills in yourself.

How EQ Makes You A Good Leader?

Research by Daniel Goleman clearly proves that you need emotional intelligence to become a great leader. The researcher states that although having technical skills and a high IQ are important to make you a good leader, you cannot become an excellent leader unless and until you have a high EQ. You can have the finest training, an analytical and incisive mind and a supply of fantastic ideas, but you won't become a great leader unless you develop a high EQ. This is because your EQ gives you the power to manipulate your emotions and that of others, and to be a good leader, you need to have the power to influence others, and if you want to improve your leadership skills and EQ at the same time, you MUST make room for mindfulness in your life.

Google, General Mills, Intel and several other renowned companies understand the importance of mindfulness and its effect on leadership skills which is why they get their employees enrolled in mindfulness based programs every year to convert them into fantastic leaders.

How Mindfulness Increases Your EQ And Leadership Potential?

Zack is a 35-year-old guy who works as a marketer in a marketing firm and aspires to become a team leader. Although he has a dream to become a good leader and eventually run his own company, he doesn't have the knack for it. He does not know how to make the best use of his emotions and make clear and fast decisions like a good leader. Since he isn't a good manager of his emotions, he lacks empathy towards others which is crucial for managing people and leading them. Moreover, he has a confused state of mind, which prevents him from becoming aware of what is required to be done. Since he lacks self-awareness, he doesn't know of his strengths and weaknesses and how to optimize the former and overcome the latter. Due to all these issues, Zack has hardly any chance of becoming a good leader like he dreams.

However, Zack has hope in mindfulness. Mindfulness makes you conscious of your state of mind, your thoughts, and beliefs, which gives you a better control of your emotions. As a result, you know what to do when, can make good decisions efficiently, are compassionate towards others and become assertive. When all these changes occur, you can automatically improve your leadership potential. To enjoy these benefits, you just need to make some time for mindfulness meditation daily.

Conclusion

We have come to the end of the book. Congratulations for reading until the end. It shows you have real commitment to transform your life positively.

I hope this book will help you build your EQ through the wonderful practice of mindfulness. Remember that you can only yield amazing results if you are consistent in your mindfulness practice, so make sure to set at least ten minutes of your time for this exercise, since it has the power to change you for the better.

Finally, if you enjoyed this book, would you be kind enough to leave a review for this book on Amazon?

If you found the book valuable, can you recommend it to others? One way to do that is to post a review on Amazon.

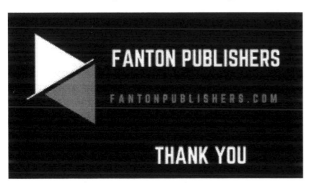

Do You Like My Book & Approach To Publishing?

If you like my writing and style and would love the ease of learning literally everything you can get your hands on from Fantonpublishers.com, I'd really need you to do me either of the following favors.

1: First, I'd Love It If You Leave a Review of This Book on Amazon.

2: Check Out My Emotional Mastery Books

Note: This list may not represent all my Keto diet books. You can check the full list by visiting my author page.

<u>Emotional Intelligence: The Mindfulness Guide To Mastering Your Emotions, Getting Ahead And Improving Your Life</u>

<u>Stress: The Psychology of Managing Pressure: Practical Strategies to turn Pressure into Positive Energy (5 Key Stress Techniques for Stress, Anxiety, and Depression Relief)</u>

<u>Failure Is Not The END: It Is An Emotional Gym: Complete Workout Plan On How To Build Your Emotional Muscle And Burning Down Anxiety To Become Emotionally Stronger, More Confident and Less Reactive</u>

<u>Subconscious Mind: Tame, Reprogram & Control Your Subconscious Mind To Transform Your Life</u>

<u>Body Language: Master Body Language: A Practical Guide to Understanding Nonverbal Communication and Improving Your Relationships</u>

<u>Shame and Guilt: Overcoming Shame and Guilt: Step By Step Guide On How to Overcome Shame and Guilt for Good</u>

<u>Anger Management: A Simple Guide on How to Deal with Anger</u>

Get updates when we publish any book that will help you master your emotions: <u>http://bit.ly/2fantonpubpersonaldevl</u>

To get a list of all my other books, please fantonwriters.com, my author central or let me send you the list by requesting them below: <u>http://bit.ly/2fantonpubnewbooks</u>

3: Grab Some Freebies On Your Way Out; Giving Is Receiving, Right?

I gave you a complimentary book at the start of the book. If you are still interested, grab it here.

<u>5 Pillar Life Transformation Checklist</u>: <u>http://bit.ly/2fantonfreebie</u>

PSS: Let Me Also Help You Save Some Money!

If you are a heavy reader, have you considered subscribing to Kindle Unlimited? You can read this and millions of other books for just $9.99 a month)! You can check it out by searching for Kindle Unlimited on Amazon!

Printed in Great Britain
by Amazon

34052710R00035